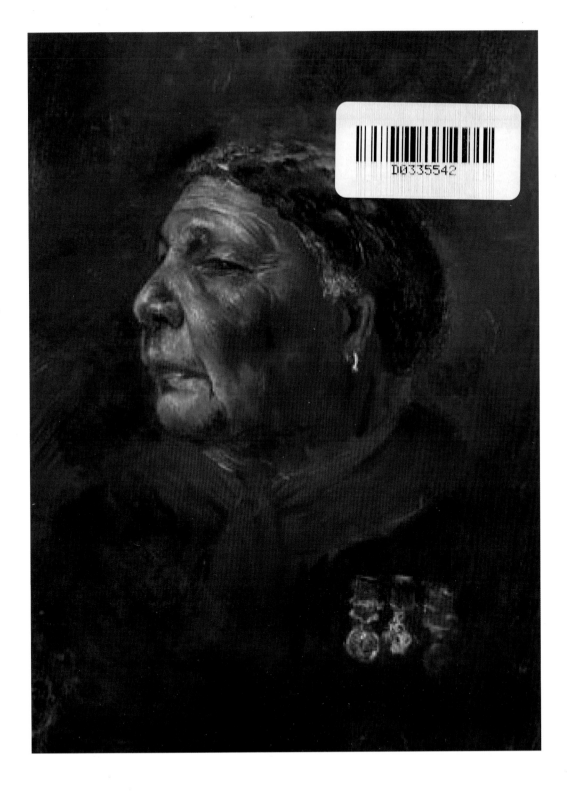

Illustrations

Front cover. A detail from the portrait of Mary Seacole by Albert Charles Challen, and a portrait of a younger Mrs Seacole reproduced courtesy of the National Library of Jamaica.

Inside back cover. *Embarkation of the sick at Balaclava*, illustrated by William Simpson, reproduced by permission of the British Library.

Previous page. The lost portrait of Mary Seacole painted in 1869 and reproduced courtesy of Helen Rappaport/National Portrait Gallery.

Page 21. A poster designed by Ralph Steadman advertising the play Black Nightingale, a production held at Oval House Theatre, London in 1989.

Page 22. Above, the new Home Office Seacole building in Marsham Street, London; below (left) the bust of Mary Seacole on display at the Royal College of Nursing headquarters in Cavendish Square, London; and below (right) Mary Seacole's grave in the Catholic cemetery in Kensal Green laid with wreaths following the memorial service of her death on 14 May 2005.

Page 23. The front cover of the 1857 autobiography *Wonderful Adventures of Mrs Seacole in Many Lands*, recently republished as a Penguin Classic.

Page 24. Images produced by the Year 5 pupils of Walnut Tree Walk School, Lambeth, London for the Florence Nightingale Museum's Mary Seacole Bicentenary London 2005 exhibition celebrating her life, work and legacy: Courtesy of the Florence Nightingale Museum, London. www.florence-nightingale.co.uk

A short history of Mary Seacole

a resource for nurses and students

Professor Elizabeth N Anionwu

RN HV Tutor PhD CBE FRCN

Acknowledgements

Sincere thanks are extended to the following for all their support and information:

- Lignum Vitae Club: Norma Mesquita.
- Mary Seacole Memorial Association: Shirley Graham-Paul, Mavis Stewart, Steve and Edita Tharpe, Dorothy Turner and Sister Monica Tywang.
- Royal College of Nursing: RCN President Sylvia Denton OBE FRCN, Katharine Collett, Drew Cullen, Emma Lang, Antonio Pineda and RCN Library staff.
- Thames Valley University Faculty of Health and Human Sciences Library staff: Margaret Buck, Lynsey Ford, Marc Forster and Pam Louison.

Thanks also to:
Ziggi Alexander; Alex Attewell, Director, Florence Nightingale Museum, London; Audrey Dewjee; Preena Gadher, Penguin Classics; Paul Kerr, October Films; Gavin McGuffie, Archivist, *Guardian* and *Observer* archive and visitor centre; Mia Morris, Well Placed Consultancy; Jane Robinson; Sam Walker, Director, Black Cultural Archives Museum, London; Marjorie Williams; Siân Evans and Eleanor Bird for editorial services; and Grey Squirrel Ltd for design and production.

Published by the Royal College of Nursing, 20 Cavendish Square, London, W1G 0RN

Publication code 002 499

ISBN 1-904114-16-4

Printed by Banbury Litho, Banbury, Oxon

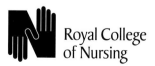

Contents

Fold-out section: About the author, the contributors, Memorial Statue Appeal.

She gave her aid to all who prayed,
To hungry, and sick and cold:
Open hand and heart, alike ready to part
Kind words, and acts, and gold.

Punch magazine, 1856

Foreword

Nurse, leader, entrepreneur and doctress; there are many labels that could be used to describe this unique and utterly absorbing figure in nursing's history - but in truth, she defies labelling. This formidable Victorian overcame innumerable hurdles - not least the innate racist attitudes of her time - to provide care for soldiers in the Crimean War, thousands of miles from her home in Jamaica.

The Royal College of Nursing celebrates the bicentenary of Mary Seacole's birth in 1805 with this accessible guide to her life, written by Professor Elizabeth Anionwu of Thames Valley University, and supplemented with thoughts from members and friends of the RCN. Although Mary was largely unappreciated in the decades following her death, we are delighted now to be able to recognise and honour her as a formidable nurse leader, alongside Florence Nightingale.

It is Mary Seacole's confidence in the pure power of nursing and her enthusiasm for delivering it that shines out and is an inspiration to nurses today. Mary carved out an important place for herself and for nursing amidst the hideous conditions of war, using as tools her natural flair for leadership, her clinical skills and above all her commitment to providing superb patient care. As this history shows, her contemporaries recognised her bravery and caring.

Dr Beverly Malone RN PhD FAAN
RCN General Secretary

Author's introduction

Professor Elizabeth Anionwu CBE FRCN
Head of the Mary Seacole Centre for Nursing Practice
Thames Valley University

Mary Seacole, nurse, herbalist, boarding house proprietor, traveller and business woman, was born in Jamaica in 1805 and died in London in 1881. She is famous for her extraordinary achievement in travelling to Turkey to care for British soldiers during the Crimean War, overcoming a lack of funds, rejection and racism along the way. Her fearlessness in attending to the troops' needs under fire, and the extent to which she was loved and respected by the men, became legendary.

Most nurses and midwives are taught about the distinguished accomplishments of Florence Nightingale during the Crimean War, but very few will have learned about Mary Seacole - despite the fact that both women were acclaimed at the time for their care and compassion to the injured and sick soldiers.

In 2005, the 200th anniversary of Mary Seacole's birth, the Royal College of Nursing (RCN) and the Mary Seacole Centre for Nursing Practice at Thames Valley University recognised the need for accessible information about Mary Seacole, for both students and qualified nurses and midwives. This short history aims to provide such an educational tool. Through it runs a Timeline, which spans 200 years from the birth of Mary Seacole in 1805 to today. This sets out a detailed chronology of Mary's life and achievements, placing them in the context of events during the Victorian era, in particular the history of Jamaica, the Crimean War, and that other great nursing icon and contemporary of Mary's, Florence Nightingale. The Timeline goes on to highlight significant events since her death.

The other part of this publication discusses Mary's achievements, and how the society of her time and of today remember her. What were the attitudes to race that affected Mary? How was she compared with Florence Nightingale?

Interspersed are short commentaries by members and friends of the RCN. At the end, you'll find a detailed reference section. If you would like to find out more about Mary Seacole and her life, start with www.maryseacole.com

Timeline

This Timeline continues over the following 16 left hand pages. It summarises the life and contribution of Mary Seacole, and reaction to her achievements from her birth in 1805 through to the present day. It sets her activities in the context of major relevant events in the Victorian period.

Sources

All information and quotations, unless otherwise referenced, are taken from the autobiography of Mary Seacole: *Wonderful Adventures of Mrs Seacole in Many Lands* which was originally published in July 1857.

Other major sources (not referenced specifically here for ease of reading) are: J Elise Gordon's 1975 article, Ziggi Alexander and Audrey Dewjee's introduction to the 1984 edition of Seacole's autobiography and Jane Robinson's 2005 study of Mary. C Woodham-Smith's biography of Florence Nightingale is also drawn on.

A woman of action

Dr Nola Ishmael OBE

The invaluable contribution that Mary Seacole made to the health care, wellbeing and comforts of soldiers fighting in the Crimea is rightfully becoming more well known. It is gratifying for those concerned with putting the record straight that the life journey of this indomitable woman is not just recognised and remembered by the more aware among nurses and other health care professionals, but also by the general public, including school children.

Mary's background prepared her in no uncertain way for the life choices she later made. From her early childhood she was curious and observant. She had a zest for learning and applied the knowledge she gained in a practical way that became her trademark in later life. She cleverly used the basic skills and knowledge gained from her mother to fuel her passion for caring. During her travels she called on that knowledge when disease and illness marked her path. She also applied what today would be described as "good old fashioned Jamaican wisdom", and developed the necessary strategies and mechanisms that would eventually help her to realise her goals. This all culminated in the history we read today.

Not for Mary the comfort of living as a genteel, Victorian woman. She saw a need and took action. She saw opportunities and maximised them. She combined caring with entrepreneurship and business acumen. Her vigour, daring and capacity for following-up and following-through supported her determination to "see, learn, plan and do", especially when the going got rough. With her innate intelligence, energy and drive that characterised her whole approach she was a woman of action who did not react but rather responded to challenge. Her style was to be proactive in situations that called for her to think strategically and to act creatively when she encountered blocks, barriers and setbacks.

The influences of the time compel us to see the difficulties that Mary experienced, but also to admire and respect the steadfastness she demonstrated and the focus she maintained as she sought to complete the mission that meant so much to

Early years

1805   Mary Seacole was born in Jamaica, then a British colony. The exact date of her birth is unknown, but the year has been assumed from her age when she died in 1881, which her death certificate recorded as 76. Mary's marriage certificate gave her maiden name as Mary Grant.

Mary's mother was a free, black Jamaican Creole, who kept a boarding house called Blundell Hall in Kingston, and also practiced as a "doctress". Mary learned some of her nursing skills and her understanding of local herbal remedies from her mother. She recalls in the opening pages of her autobiography how: "It was very natural that I should inherit her tastes; and so I had from early youth a yearning for medical knowledge and practice which has never deserted me. ...and I was very young when I began to make use of the little knowledge I had acquired from watching my mother, upon a great sufferer – my doll. ...and whatever disease was most prevalent in Kingston, be sure my poor doll soon contracted it."

Very little is known about Mary's father, except that he was a Scottish soldier, although recent research by Robinson (2005) has uncovered a man who could have been this father, an officer called James Grant. Mary had a sister, Louisa, and a brother, Edward.

Mary's autobiography recounts how as a young child, she was looked after by an old lady who brought her up as though one of her grandchildren. She still saw her mother frequently. She also describes how she travelled to England with relatives, probably when she was in her teens, and stayed there for about a year. Mary recalls that she and her companion were taunted about the colour of their skin by young children in a London street.

1807   The Slave Trade Act outlawed involvement of British ships in trading slaves from Africa.

1820   Florence Nightingale was born in Florence, Italy, on 12 May.

her. Today, her resoluteness and firm conviction can only be aspired to. Gaining acceptance from the authority of the day was her hope - receiving recognition and having her memory immortalised by future generations is her ultimate reward.

The Timeline draws the reader to visualise the events that captured the headlines of the day, as they happened. It brings together an orderly account of an inspirational leader of the nineteenth century whose time has finally come. It fills in the gaps and clears up much of the speculation of Mary's later years.

Professor Elizabeth Anionwu and the RCN are to be congratulated for bringing this well researched publication to our attention. It is an honour to be associated with this work.

1823   Around this time, Mary travelled to London again, this time on her own. She took with her a large amount of West Indian pickles and preserves to sell. Mary writes about other voyages too, though gives no dates, to New Providence in the Bahamas, Cuba and Haiti (then named Saint-Domingue).

Learning her trade

1826   Mary returned to Jamaica after her second visit to Britain. Over the next decade, she nursed her patroness right through to the final illness. Mary then lived at Blundell Hall, helping her mother care for soldiers recovering from yellow fever.

1833   The Abolition of Slavery Act made slavery in the British Empire illegal.

1836   Mary married Englishman Edwin Horatio Hamilton Seacole on 10 November - his name is given as on his baptism registration of 18 September 1803 (Robinson, 2005a). Immediately following the wedding, they returned to the Jamaican district of Black Rivers and set up a store.

   Mary provides no details of how she first met her husband. Seacole is described as a merchant in Mary's will, and was already in delicate health at the time of their marriage. He was probably born in Prittlewell, Essex, and was Godson of Viscount Nelson, the British naval hero (Seacole, 1876). Robinson (2005) records the fascinating Seacole family legend that Edwin's father, a "surgeon, apothecary, and man midwife", first forged a connection with Nelson at the time of the second pregnancy of Nelson's mistress, Lady Hamilton.

1838   All slaves in Jamaica were emancipated on 1 August. They were now known as "full free". This followed the limited emancipation of slaves announced in August 1834 (National Library of Jamaica).

Attitudes to race in Victorian Britain

Colonial rule

Attitudes to race in Victorian Britain were complex, shifting and divergent. The reign of Queen Victoria (1837-1901) began just after the Act to abolish slavery in 1833. It witnessed both the expansion of the Empire, and significant local opposition to British rule which led to brutal suppression. In the 1865 Morant Bay Rebellion in Jamaica, for example, leaders of the uprising Paul Bogle and George William Gordon were hanged, and nearly 450 others were killed. A further 600 people were flogged, some before being put to death. The middle classes of Britain were whipped into a frenzy of fear about such uprisings as this and the Indian Rebellion of 1857, while others were horrified by the nature of the suppression. The Morant Bay Rebellion led to a major debate in Britain, with opinion for and against Edward Eyre, the British Governor of Jamaica, who was ultimately recalled. The end of the Victorian era came a year after the convening of the first ever Pan-African Conference, held in London in 1900. This heralded the emergence of a powerful movement for independence from colonial rule.

Racist attitudes

The arguments that raged around slavery and the British Empire primarily centred on whether black people could really be considered on an equal status with whites. Powerful economic forces influenced some of those who wanted to maintain the status quo and retain the immensely profitable outcomes, whether from slavery or from an Empire that depended on a "native" workforce. "Scientific racism" set out arguments to support theories of white racial superiority. Some opinions were deeply offensive and likened the "Negro" to something nearer to an animal than a human being. Some people expressed abhorrence of relationships between different ethnic groups and called for them to be outlawed.

Throughout this period there were also forces opposed to such racist notions. Historians describe the sharply contrasting and strongly articulated views that

1843 Blundell Hall burned down in the great fire that devastated Kingston. New Blundell Hall was then constructed at 7 East Street, Kingston.

1844 Mary's husband became more frail: "I kept him alive by kind nursing and attention as long as I could." When he deteriorated, they came back to New Blundell Hall and he died in October of this year, one month after their return. Mary "felt it bitterly". Soon after she also lost her mother.

1850 Mary nursed victims of the Kingston cholera epidemic. She acknowledged receiving advice about treating the condition from a doctor lodging at New Blundell Hall.

Meanwhile, in July, Florence Nightingale made a trip, lasting for two weeks, to the Kaiserswerth Institute in Germany, which incorporated an infant school, orphanage and a hospital. The following year, she made another, three-month visit.

1851 It was probably in this year that Mary made the arduous voyage to Cruces, a gold prospecting town in Panama (then called New Granada), to visit her brother Edward, who had recently left Jamaica to set up the Independent Hotel. Mary later wrote: "...I made money rapidly, and pressed my brother to return to Kingston. Poor fellow! It would have been well for him had he done so; for he stayed only to find a grave on the Isthmus of Panama."

In Cruces, Mary ended up coping virtually single-handedly with a cholera epidemic, when it all became too much for a local dentist and a Spanish doctor - Mary commented in her autobiography: "I think their chief reliance was on the yellow woman from Jamaica with the cholera medicine." Mary even carried out a post-mortem on a child of barely a year old who had died of cholera. Mary herself survived a bout of the illness. She went on to renovate a building, which she was to call the British Hotel, a non-residential catering establishment with an adjacent barber's shop.

were held by writers, scientists, religious leaders, politicians, the media and sections of the general public (e.g. Fryer, 1984; Wilson, 2003). They provide a context to explain how racism may well have played a part in why Mary Seacole, and two other black Caribbean nurses we know about, were not invited to go to the Crimea (Public Record Office).

Seacole's experience

Mary Seacole herself is sometimes dismissive of both those darker than herself as well as her fellow Jamaican Creoles. The term "Creole" has various meanings, one of which describes people of mixed black and European descent. While extremely proud of her Scottish heritage, Mary was also very forthright in her rejection of any person expressing sentiments of white superiority. She recounts how at an American Independence reception in Panama, a sallow, tobacco-chewing American included the following in his toast to her: "…I calculate, gentlemen, you're all as vexed as I am that she's not wholly white, but I du reckon on your rejoicing with me that she's so many shades removed from being entirely black; and I guess, if we could bleach her by any means we would; and thus make her acceptable in any company as she deserves to be. Gentlemen, I give you Aunty Seacole." She includes in her response "…and as to his offer of bleaching me, I should, even if it were practicable, decline it without any thanks. As to the society which the process might gain me admission into, all I can say is, that, judging from the specimens I have met with here and elsewhere, I don't think that I shall lose much by being excluded from it. So, gentlemen, I drink to you and the general reformation of American manners."

McKenna (1997) and Frederick (2003) have analysed Mary's seemingly contradictory views about race and identity. Her conflicting attitudes are best understood within the context of the complex factors impacting on Jamaican Creole society. Out of the harsh system of slavery developed powerful hierarchies favouring those of a lighter shade of skin colour. In addition, Mary was primarily writing for an English audience which is why she may have focused more on racial discrimination in North America.

Mary acknowledges in her autobiography that it was through her Creole heritage that she learned the "healing art". But she could see that it was these very origins that may have been at the root of her repeated rejection in 1854, when she tried to offer her nursing services to the authorities responsible for the troops in the Crimea. She writes that she was "so certain of the service I could render among the sick soldiery, and yet I found it so difficult to convince others of these facts. Doubts and suspicions arose in my heart for the first and last time, thank Heaven. Was it possible that American prejudices against colour had some root

1853   Mary cared for victims of a yellow fever epidemic in Jamaica. She was invited by the medical authorities to supervise nursing services at Up-Park Camp in Kingston, headquarters of the British Army. Mary reorganised New Blundell Hall to function as a hospital to care for her patients. She formed strong maternal attachments to these soldiers, and her feelings for them later drove her to the Crimea.

Although in her autobiography Mary is sometimes negative about her fellow Creoles, when writing about this period she does acknowledge that her expertise in herbalism was due to this heritage: "...another benefit has been conferred upon them by inclining the Creoles to practise the healing art, and inducing them to seek out the simple remedies which are available for the terrible diseases by which foreigners are attacked, and which are found growing under the same circumstances which produce the ills they minister to. So true is it, that beside the nettle ever grows the cure for its sting."

Thousands of miles away in the Crimean Peninsula, conflict broke out when Turkey declared war on Russia (Kerr et al., 2000; Ponting, 2004).

The Crimean War

1854   England and France joined forces with Turkey against Russia.

On 21 October, Florence Nightingale left London for Scutari, accompanied by 38 nurses. She arrived at the Barrack Hospital on 5 November. Scutari (now called Uskudar) is located at the mouth of the Bosphorus, at the south of the Black Sea, and wounded troops were brought here from the centre of the war on the Crimean Peninsula, several hundred miles away.

Mary left Jamaica in the spring in order to wind up outstanding issues about her hotel and returned to Panama's Navy Bay (now known as Colon). She then travelled to England, where she planned to pursue some

here? Did these ladies shrink from accepting my aid because my blood flowed beneath a somewhat duskier skin than theirs?"

There are other examples of racial prejudice towards nurses who wanted to go to the Crimea cited in recent historical studies (Alexander, 1990; Kerr et al, 2000). "A certain Miss Belgrave was rejected because a 'West Indian constitution is not the one best able to bear the fatigue of nursing …though Mrs B looks robust – and some English patients would object to a nurse being so nearly a person of color [sic]'. " Similarly, Elizabeth Purcell, who was first described as an "exemplary character", was then rejected at fifty-two, some ten years younger than many of the nurses who went out to the Crimea, for being "too old and almost black" (Public Record Office).

claims in a Panamanian mining company. However, before she left Jamaica, Mary heard that war has been declared against Russia, and she decided to combine her original aim with a plan to enlist as a nurse in the Crimea. She wrote: "Now, no sooner had I heard of war somewhere, than I longed to witness it; and when I was told that many of the regiments I had known so well in Jamaica had left England for the scene of action, the desire to join them became stronger than ever."

Mary arrived in London in the autumn of 1854, just after the Battle of Alma had been fought on 20 September. She came armed with glowing testimonials, including one from the medical officer of a Panamanian gold-mining company, who had "had many opportunities of witnessing her professional zeal and ability in the treatment of aggravated forms of tropical diseases".

Mary began repeatedly offering her services to care for troops in the Crimea, but in vain. She approached the War Office, the Quartermaster-General's Department, the Medical Department and "Mrs H" (Elizabeth Herbert, wife of Sidney Herbert, Secretary at War), who was in charge of the campaign to recruit a second group of nurses to join Florence Nightingale in Scutari.

Finally, Mary applied to the managers of the Crimean Fund to secure a passage to the war zone, but once more experienced rejection. This rebuff seemed to leave her heartbroken and wondering whether racism was at work in England. "The disappointment seemed a cruel one. I felt certain of the service I could render among the sick soldiery," she writes, "and yet I found it so difficult to convince others of these facts. Doubts and suspicions arose in my heart for the first and last time, thank Heaven. Was it possible that American prejudices against colour had some root here?" Her disappointment is such that: "Tears streamed down my foolish cheeks, as I stood in the fast thinning streets; tears of grief that any should doubt my motives – that Heaven should deny me the opportunity that I sought. Then I stood still, and looking upward

An inclusive profession

RCN President Sylvia Denton OBE FRCN

As a practising nurse myself, I have been inspired and informed by Mary Seacole's example. Nurses are the backbone of the health care workforce, yet we have always had to work hard to get our messages across and have our work properly valued. Understanding how Mary rose to the challenges is an inspiration to us all.

Today, we understand as nurses that we have to work in partnership with our patients and their families. But the finest nurses, like Mary Seacole, have always done that, as we can see from the accounts of how warmly her patients liked and respected her.

As a symbol of diversity, Mary Seacole has a special significance for black and minority ethnic nurses. I am proud to have played my part in advocating that diversity is strength and not a weakness. Everyone in the nursing family deserves to be treated with respect as a valuable member of the team. We cannot afford to have anyone leaving nursing because they feel excluded or discriminated against.

Mary had to take on the Establishment just because she wanted to care for wounded British soldiers in the Crimea. We have to make sure that nursing today is a welcoming and inclusive profession because society needs nurses – and still there are not enough of us.

It is wonderful that Mary Seacole has recently been recognised for her outstanding role in Britain's and nursing's history by being voted the greatest black Briton. What a wonderful demonstration of public affection and respect. For the last ten years, the Department of Health has been awarding scholarships in her name, valuing the work of black and minority ethnic nurses. The pioneering work done by the modern Mary Seacole scholars has been making a real difference to

through and through the dark clouds that shadowed London, prayed aloud for help."

1855   Mary, now in her fiftieth year, refused to be thwarted in realising her dream of caring for the British soldiers. She decided to fund her own passage to the Crimea. She also purchased medicines and home comforts that she thought would be useful for the military. To alert her friends in Sevastopol, Mary dispatched printed cards announcing that she would be setting sail for Balaclava on 25 January, on the screw-steamer *Hollander*.

During this time, she met up again with a relative of her late husband, a Mr Thomas Day, who was bound for Balaclava to attend to some shipping business. The two decided to operate as "sutlers", people selling food and drink to soldiers - forerunners to official army catering services such as the Navy, Army, and Air Force Institutes (NAAFI). To this end, they established the firm of Seacole and Day, which would operate a store and a hotel in a location near the army camp outside Balaclava.

Mary arrived in Turkey in March 1855 and, ever the networker, left the ship armed with a letter of introduction to Florence Nightingale, given to her by a fellow-passenger, a doctor she had known in Jamaica. At the Barrack Hospital in Scutari, a sergeant from Jamaica recognised Mary and escorted her on a tour of the wards, which "rendered it unnecessary for me to trouble the busy nurses". Other soldiers recognised Mary and she spent the day sitting by their beds trying to cheer them up, even adjusting some of their bandages. While she waited to see Florence Nightingale, Mary recounts in her autobiography that she encountered and was quizzed by Florence's companion, Mrs Selina Bracebridge: *I fancy Mrs B thought that I sought for employment at Scutari, for she said very kindly "Miss Nightingale has the entire management of our hospital staff, but I do not think that any vacancy." "Excuse me, ma'am," I interrupt her with, "but I am bound for the front in a few days," and my questioner leaves me more surprised than ever.*

patient care. I know that Mary, like me, would be proud of the nurses of today - nurses like Elizabeth Anionwu, whose contribution to nursing and patient care includes her work in highlighting Mary Seacole's life and achievements.

I am honoured to be leading the RCN's support for the campaign to have a memorial to Mary Seacole in London, both with my practical support and by using my influence as RCN President. Leadership is about action, not position, and diversity is one of the major themes of my presidency.

Mary's emergence from the shadows of history has been helped by the discovery of a previously unknown portrait of her. We are very grateful to Helen Rappaport and the National Portrait Gallery for their permission to reproduce the newly-found portrait in this publication. What a role model she is - that warm hearted, intelligent, determined and expert nurse. We can all learn from Mary Seacole's example, and this publication is designed to help you do just that.

Mary's autobiography describes her brief meeting with Florence Nightingale, and how Florence arranged overnight accommodation for her in the washerwomen's quarters. As a footnote in Chapter 9 Mary notes, without further details, that, "Subsequently I saw much of Miss Nightingale, at Balaclava".

By around July 1855, Mary and Mr Day had organised the building of the British Hotel near Balaclava on the Crimean Peninsula. It was located on Spring Hill, just beyond Kadikoi, near a hill known as the "Col". The hotel provided soldiers of all ranks with accommodation, food, other provisions and nursing care. References by some men who provided testaments in Mary's autobiography, including John Hall, Inspector-General of Hospitals in the Crimea, show this care included Creole herbal remedies. Among visitors at the hotel was Alexis Benoît Soyer, the French chef who became renowned for his voluntary efforts to improve the quality of food for the British soldiers. In the early summer of 1855, he describes his first meeting with "the celebrated Mrs Seacole" at the hotel, where she invited him to take a glass of champagne with a Major-General Sir John Campbell (Soyer, 1995 edition). In September, after the fall of Sevastopol, Mary was one of the first women to enter the city from the English lines.

1856   Mary sets out in great detail the nourishment and care she provided for the wounded and sick soldiers, regardless of which side they were on. Her book also contains many testimonies from those she nursed and supported during the dark days of war. There are also independently published accounts from journalists, doctors, military personnel and others who visited the battlefields, recognising her skills, compassion and hard work on behalf of the victims of war (examples quoted in this publication are cited in Gordon, 1975; Alexander and Dewjee, 1984; Robinson, 2005; Salih, 2005).

Among the most influential of commentators was Sir William Howard Russell, the celebrated war correspondent of *The Times* newspaper. His vivid and uncensored dispatches helped alert the British public to the desperate conditions experienced by ordinary soldiers (Kerr et al, 2000; Ponting, 2004). On 11

Keeping the memory alive

"This is wonderful news. As a black Jamaican woman in the 19th century, Mary Seacole stood up against the discrimination and prejudices she encountered. The RCN and I believe that Mary Seacole deserves a statue in London to commemorate her important place in Britain's nursing history."
Sylvia Denton, OBE FRCN, RCN President, quoted in *The Times*, 10 February 2004, following the announcement that Mary Seacole had come first in an online vote to find the greatest black Briton (Young, 2004).

Two hundred years after her birth, Mary Seacole appears at last to have gained a more secure footing in the annals of nursing history. The Timeline demonstrates that Mary's contemporaries had already acknowledged the immense contribution she made as a nurse. She had a high public profile, and her achievements were greatly celebrated - as poignantly illustrated by Sir William H Russell, *The Times* war correspondent, in his foreword to the 1857 edition of her autobiography: "I should have thought that no preface would have been required to introduce Mrs. Seacole to the British public, …I trust that England will not forget one who nursed her sick, who sought out her wounded to aid and succour them, and who performed the last offices for some of her illustrious dead."

Regardless of these fine sentiments, Mary Seacole did fade into virtual obscurity in Britain for nearly a century following her death in 1881. There were glimmers of interest in the mid-twentieth century – Helen Rappaport (2005) makes reference to a 1954 article in *The Times* in which a journalist concluded that Seacole's work "might serve as a great example to the many West Indian nurses who now receive a better training than Mrs Seacole gathered from her mother".

In Jamaica, Mary's memory was kept alive for much longer. For example, the important role played by the Kingston-based Jamaican Nurses' Association

April 1857 he recalled: "I have seen [Mrs Seacole] go down, under fire with her little store of creature comforts for our wounded men; and a more tender or skilful hand about a wound or a broken limb could not be found amongst our best surgeons. I saw her at the assaults on the Redan, at the Battle of Tchernaya, at the fall of Sebastopol, laden ...with wine, bandages and food for the wounded or the prisoners. Her hands, too, performed the last offices for some of the noblest of our slain."

In March, the war suddenly ended. Mary found herself in severe financial difficulties as recently purchased stores were now redundant and many personal accounts had not been settled. Despite this, in July *The Illustrated London News* noted her presence at a ceremony to mark the official departure of troops from The Crimea: "Conspicuous in the foreground, Mrs Seacole, dressed in a plaid riding-habit, and the smartest of hats, calling everybody her son. She was very much liked."

In contrast, Florence Nightingale left the Crimea for England in July determined to avoid the planned fanfare. C Woodham-Smith writes that Florence was "obsessed by a sense of failure. In fact, in the midst of the muddle and the filth, the agony and the defeats, she had brought about a revolution".

By 26 August, Mary was back in London, and her guest appearance at a "Dinner to the Guards" at the Royal Surrey Gardens was recorded in *The Times*.

The aftermath of war

On 28 October 1856 the *London Gazette* featured a notice petitioning for bankruptcy proceedings against Mary Seacole and Thomas Day. On 6 November, the official hearing took place at the Bankruptcy Court in London's Basinghall Street. *The Times* published several letters from well wishers who, hearing of her plight, wanted to establish a fund for Mary. They included Captain Hussey Fane Keane, Major-General Lord Rokeby and Sir William

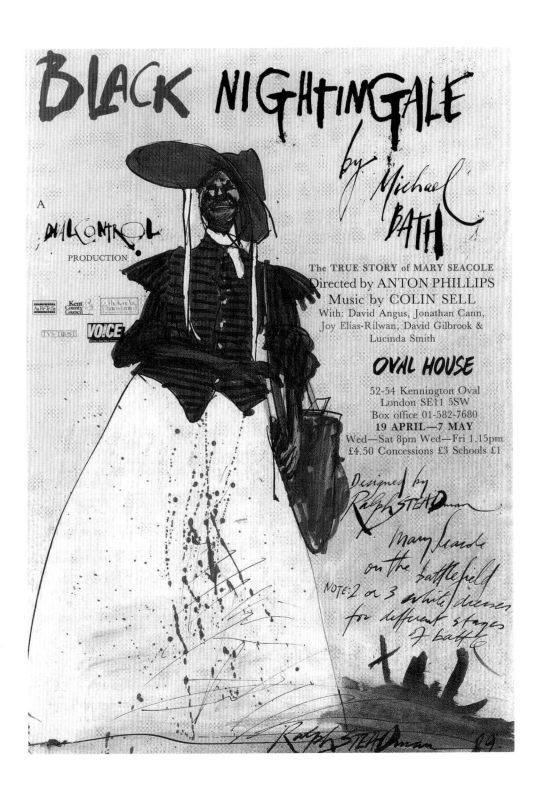

BLACK NIGHTINGALE

by Michael **BATH**

A **DIAL CONTROL** PRODUCTION

The **TRUE STORY** of MARY SEACOLE
Directed by ANTON PHILLIPS
Music by COLIN SELL
With: David Angus, Jonathan Cann,
Joy Elias-Rilwan, David Gilbrook &
Lucinda Smith

OVAL HOUSE

52-54 Kennington Oval
London SE11 5SW
Box office 01-582-7680
19 APRIL—7 MAY
Wed—Sat 8pm Wed—Fri 1.15pm
£4.50 Concessions £3 Schools £1

Designed by
Ralph STEADman

Mary Seacole
on the battlefield
NOTE: 2 or 3 white dresses
for different stages
of battle

Ralph STEADman 89.

21

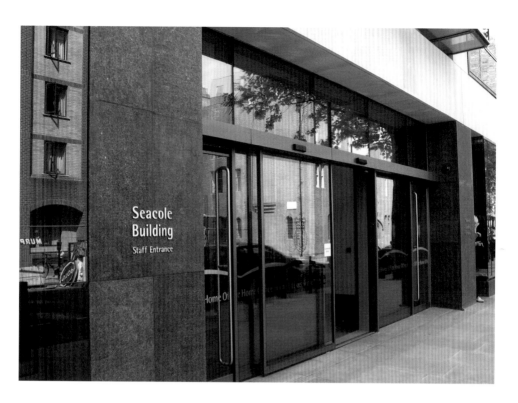

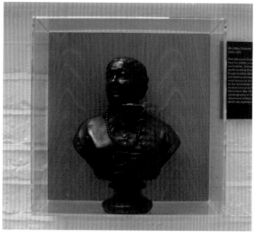

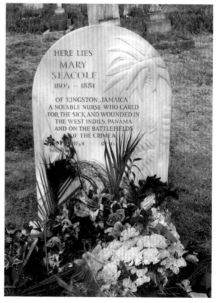

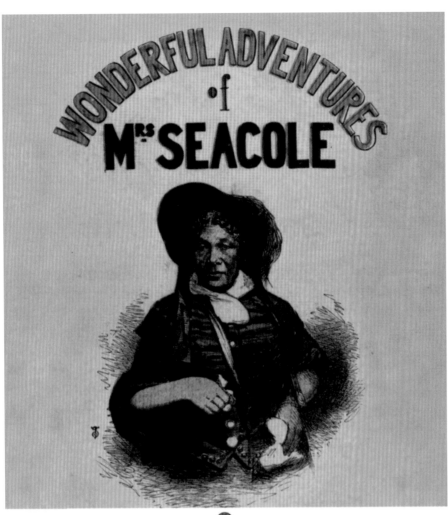

PENGUIN CLASSICS

MARY SEACOLE

*Wonderful Adventures of Mrs Seacole
in Many Lands*

The Florence Nightingale Museum was keen to engage the local community in their exhibition "The Wonderful Mrs Seacole", and approached The Walnut Tree Walk School. The Year 5 pupils already had some knowledge of Mary Seacole after learning about her in the National Curriculum. The children's words and drawings show that Mary Seacole is a worthy role model for us today.

**Mary Seacole Bicentenary
London 2005**

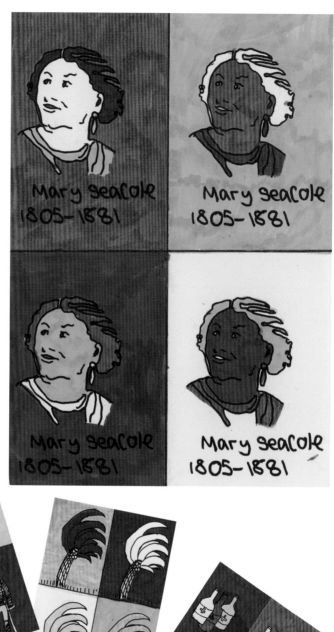

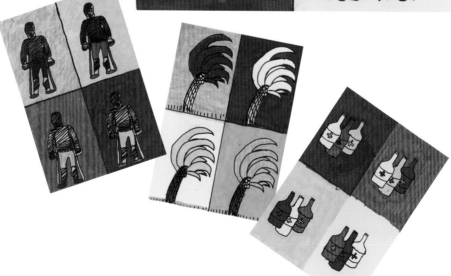

merits wider recognition. In 1954, the association named their new headquarters, which opened in 1960, Mary Seacole House; and members such as Mary Seivwright (1961), Cynthia Vernon (1969), Edna Tulloch (1971) and Eileen Cootes-Peterkin (1961, 1961a) all published articles about Mary Seacole in nursing journals.

Comparing coverage with Florence Nightingale

Given their joint reputation in the nineteenth century, one wonders why nursing literature has until recently had such meagre reference to Mary Seacole, in comparison with Florence Nightingale? A rudimentary measure of this disparity compares the number of articles in past issues of nursing journals (as recorded in the Royal College of Nursing Bibliography of Nursing Literature; Thompson, 1968, 1974; Walsh, 1985, 1986). The results make interesting reading (and could be the subject of further investigations for those interested in the way our profession's history is recorded). Between 1859 and 1980, the start of the decade that saw a wave of interest with the reprinting of Mary's autobiography, only three of 97 relevant publications are related to Mary Seacole (and one of these is not recorded in the index). This contrasts to 94 for Florence Nightingale.

Table 1:

Number of references to Florence Nightingale and Mary Seacole in the RCN's Bibliography of Nursing Literature during the period 1859 and 1980.

Period	1859-1960	1961-1970	1971-1975	1976-1980	Total
Florence Nightingale	50	16	13	15	94 (97%)
Mary Seacole	1[1]	1[2]	1[3]	0	3 (3%)
Total	51	17	14	15	97 (100%)

1. Black (1943) 2. Seivwright (1961) 3. Gordon (1975)

Howard Russell. In December *Punch* magazine supported the Seacole Fund by publishing a poem, *A Stir for Seacole* (to be sung to the tune of the nursery rhyme *Old King Cole*). The poem concluded:

"She gave her aid to all who prayed,
To hungry, and sick and cold:
Open hand and heart, alike ready to part
Kind words, and acts, and gold.
And now the good soul is 'in the hole',
What red-coat in all the land,
But to set her upon her legs again
Will not lend a willing hand?"

1857 In February the courts declared Mary no longer a debtor. She went on to publish a best-selling autobiography that summer, entitled *Wonderful Adventures of Mrs Seacole in Many Lands (see page 23)*. It went into a second edition within a year.

Mary became increasingly celebrated. *Punch* magazine published further articles and a cartoon about her, and a four-day gala was held in her honour during July, at the Royal Surrey Gardens in London. Unfortunately, for various reasons, the gala only raised £228 for Mary. During the next two years, Mary travelled around the country visiting military hospitals and barracks.

1858 During a visit to Jamaica, the novelist Anthony Trollope stayed at New Blundell Hall and later wrote (Trollope, 1859) about the landlady Louisa, Mary's sister. Louisa was obviously proud of Mary, and told Trollope that Mary had wanted to go in 1857 to India with the Army who were fighting the Indian Rebellion, but that Queen Victoria would not let her because her life was "too precious".

1859 Henry Weekes sculpted a bust of Mary Seacole that is now housed in the Getty Museum (Getty Museum, Los Angeles).

Mary left for Jamaica where, evidence suggests, she remained until 1865 (Rappaport, 2005).

New interest

The good news is the significant interest in Mary Seacole now being shown by the nursing profession within the UK. Her enhanced profile "…comes at a time when the NHS and the profession are trying to eradicate racism and discrimination, and encourage the promotion of people on their merit. If Mary were here today, she would say that is what should happen. She would not put up with discrimination" (Pearce, 2004). This level of awareness could not have happened without the initial efforts of many people and organisations, nursing and non-nursing alike, such as J Elise Gordon, Ziggi Alexander, Audrey Dewjee and UK-based organisations such as the Lignum Vitae, Jamaican Nurses' Association and the Mary Seacole Memorial Association.

It is, therefore, extremely sad and a disservice to those who've fought for Mary's place in history, to read: "The final irony is that, as Nightingale's star wanes, the post-colonial atmosphere of political correctness has now ensured that Mary Seacole's will once more burn bright" (Rappaport, 2005).

Florence Nightingale's star is far from waning; her contribution is kept much alive by an excellent museum. The museum's website (www.florence-nightingale. co.uk) shows a healthy number of recent biographies (Gill, 2004; Small, 1998) and Mark Bostridge is writing another. Another recent book (Dossey et al., 2005) discusses the relevance of Florence Nightingale to modern day health care. During the period 1982-2004 the Cumulative Index to Nursing & Allied Health Literature (CINAHL) cites 204 articles that contain Florence Nightingale in the title. A minority of these do not sing her praises. Compare this to the total of 27 titles containing Mary Seacole.

The years 2004 to 2005 witnessed the start of a colossal increase in the national profile of Mary Seacole due to extensive media coverage. The triggers were a campaign for a statue of her in central London (Duffin, 2004), coming first in the 100 Great Black Britons online competition (Taylor, 2004) and the announcement of the discovery of a lost portrait (*Nursing Standard*, 2005; and see reference for *Portrait*).

1860   Florence Nightingale published *Notes on Nursing. What it is, and What it is Not* (Nightingale, 1860). The Nightingale Training School for nurses at St Thomas' Hospital, London, was established. It was funded from public subscriptions made to the Nightingale Fund, which had been launched in 1855 to enable the nation to demonstrate gratitude to Nightingale for her efforts during the Crimean War.

Later years

1865   The Morant Bay Rebellion against British rule in Jamaica. The uprising was led by Paul Bogle and George William Gordon, who were both hanged, and over 400 others were killed in its suppression (Fryer, 1984). Mary may well have been in Jamaica at the time.

1867   Mary was by now back in England. Her fame continued, but so did her financial troubles. Another fund was established to support her, this time with the public backing of Queen Victoria.

1869   Mary's portrait was painted by Albert Charles Challen. The picture was lost for many years, but was unearthed in 2002 by historian Helen Rappaport (Rappaport, 2005), who loaned it to the National Portrait Gallery. There it has been on display since January 2005.

1871   The sculptor Count Gleichen, half-nephew of Queen Victoria, made a terracotta bust of Mary. It was exhibited at the Summer Exhibition of the Royal Academy in 1872 and is now located in the Institute of Jamaica.

1873   Mary had become masseuse to the Princess of Wales, who suffered from a rheumatic knee, although there is little documentary evidence about how this appointment came about. The only known photograph of Mary Seacole, printed on a visiting card, was taken around this period (Robinson, 2005). Her final years were divided between Jamaica and England. Wherever she was, there are accounts that Mary was acknowledged in public and she received a continuous flow of visitors.

Seacole and Nightingale

Many of the first writers reviving Mary Seacole's memory describe her as the "Florence Nightingale of Jamaica", a pattern followed by more recent publications and online articles (Gustafson, 1996; Messmer and Parchment, 1996; Seaton, 2002). No such comparative description, however well-intentioned, is required; while there were some similarities between Florence and Mary, they should both be acclaimed for their very different achievements in nursing. It is a disservice to Mary Seacole to set her in the shadow of Florence Nightingale by calling her the "Black Nightingale".

These two nursing luminaries had very different approaches to their task, though they both saw themselves as a mother figure to the soldiers (Gill, 2004). As historian A N Wilson points out: "Florence Nightingale's admirable hospital was several hundred miles from the Crimean peninsula. Mary Seacole did not pretend to Nightingale's formidable gifts of organisation, but she was in the very front line. Her British hotel in Balaclava was an important refuge. …The ranks who had a fear of hospitals felt more at ease with Mother Seacole than in the Turkish field hospitals" (Wilson, 2003). Bostridge (2004) argues that "while there is every reason to commemorate her remarkable contribution to nursing, the comparison with Nightingale does justice to neither. There is no doubt that in terms of practical nursing expertise, Seacole far outdistanced Nightingale's experience. Her work included preparing medicines, diagnosis and minor surgery, and she describes carrying out her 'first and last' postmortem, on a baby, to learn more about cholera".

What did they think of each other?

Infuriatingly, despite their dual fame during the Crimean War, there is a dearth of historical documents or published comments about the relationship between the two nursing icons. How often did they meet and what did they really think of each other? Mary recalls seeing much of Florence in Balaclava, but she provided no further details. She did, however, chronicle her impressions of their

1881   Mary Seacole became ill in April, and died in London on 14 May. The cause of her death was registered as "Apoplexy 16 days Coma 3 days". In her will Mary stated: "I desire to be buried in the Catholic portion of the Cemetery at Kensal Green, otherwise known as St Mary's Catholic Cemetery in Harrow Road, London" (Seacole, 1876). Her grave there is number 5816. Mary's estate was valued at a total of £2,615.11s.7d, to be distributed among family and friends. This was a significant amount of money for the time and makes clear that at the time of her death, Mary had recovered from her earlier financial troubles.

Obituaries and notices of Mary's death appeared in newspapers such as *The Times* (24 May), *The Manchester Guardian* (23 May) and the Jamaican *Daily Gleaner* (9 June), which reported that Mary had been awarded "English, French, Russian and Turkish decorations" (Robinson, 2005; McGuffie, 2004; Alexander and Dewjee, 1984). Mystery surrounds these medals, as their nature and current whereabouts is unknown. Some historians have suggested they may have been dress medals or miniatures, while others have identified two as the Turkish Order of the Mejidie and the French Legion of Honour (Alexander and Dewjee, 1984; Robinson, 2005; Salih, 2005).

1905   Mary's sister Louisa Grant died in Jamaica at the age of 90.

Renewed recognition

1907   Florence Nightingale was awarded the Order of Merit, in addition to previous international honours.

1910   Florence Nightingale died in London on 13 August, aged 90 years.

1915   The Crimean War Memorial was erected In London near the junction of Lower Regent Street and Pall Mall. It included a statue of Florence Nightingale but not one of Mary Seacole (Anionwu, 2003). This indifference to Mary's achievements continued for much of the first half of the twentieth century.

first acquaintance: "…standing thus in repose, and yet keenly observant – the greatest sign of impatience at any time a slight, perhaps unwitting motion of the right foot – was Florence Nightingale – that English woman whose name shall never die, but sound like music on the lips of British men until the hour of doom."

In contrast, Florence Nightingale seemed to have very mixed feelings about Mary Seacole, judging from remarks in a letter to her brother-in-law Sir Harry Verney MP, in August 1870 (Nightingale, 1870 cited in Alexander, 1990; Salih, 2005; Robinson, 2005). Florence seems to have been asked for her views on Mary, and she made it clear that she did not want these made public: the relevant page is headed "Burn". She writes: "Mrs Seacole. I dare say you know more about her than I do. She kept – I will not call it a 'bad house' but something not very unlike it in the Crimean War. She was very kind to the men &, what is more, to the Officers - & did some good - & made many drunk. (A shameful ignorant imposture was practised on the Queen who subscribed to the 'Seacole testimonial'). I had the greatest difficulty in repelling Mrs Seacole's advances, & in preventing association between her & my nurses (absolutely out of the question) when we established 2 hospitals nursed by us between Kadikoi & the 'Seacole Establishment' in the Crimea" (Robinson, 2005).

The letter makes clear her concerns about royal involvement with the Seacole Fund.

Helen Rappaport (2005) notes that no record seems to exist of Queen Victoria ever having extended an invitation to meet Mary Seacole. She wonders whether Florence Nightingale, whom the Queen greatly revered, might have influenced this situation; Florence may have been disdainful of Mary's "bad house" and her sense of propriety offended by the serving of alcohol in this establishment. It is well recognised that Florence wished to transform the contemporary image of nursing, so negatively depicted in Charles Dickens' novel *Martin Chuzzlewit*, with its unkempt and dissolute nurses, Sarah Gamp and Betsy Prig.

It is difficult to determine how much Florence's opinions were influenced by Mary's different ethnic and cultural background and social class. Mary certainly believed Florence had a good opinion about her - the chef Alexis Soyer (1857) recorded how Mary had told him at least 20 times that Florence Nightingale was very fond of her and had provided board and lodging for Mary in Scutari. When he visited the Land Transport Corps Hospital, Soyer passed on Mary's greetings to Florence, who, he recounts, replied with a smile: "I should like to see her before she leaves, as I hear she has done a great deal of good for the poor soldiers."

1947　J A Rogers devoted a chapter to Mary Seacole in his landmark book on significant people of African descent (Rogers, 1947).

1954　The centenary of British involvement in the Crimean War. Jamaica formally recognised Mary Seacole in various ways: the Jamaican General Trained Nurses' Association (now the Jamaican Nurses' Association) decided to name their proposed Kingston headquarters Mary Seacole House (this was opened in 1960); a ward in Kingston Public Hospital was also named after Mary Seacole in 1956 (Williams M, 2005), and a residence at the University of the West Indies was named Seacole Hall in 1957 (University of the West Indies, 1985).

1961　An article in *The Jamaican Nurse* noted that some reports say Mary died in Kingston, others in London, and that her final resting place is unknown and unmarked. It also detailed six Jamaican references between 1905 and 1951 to Mary Seacole, in articles, newspapers and a radio broadcast (Seivwright, 1961).

1962　Jamaica became independent from Britain on 6 August (National Library of Jamaica).

1973　By now, the decaying grave of Mary Seacole had been located at Kensal Green through a chance discovery by the journalist and editor of the *Nursing Mirror*, J Elise Gordon. In a copy of Mary's autobiography, Gordon found a slip of paper which made reference to Mary's will (Seacole, 1876), where she had stated where she wanted to be buried (Gordon, 1975; *Nursing Mirror*, 1977; *Jamaican Nurse*, 1973; Tywang, 2004).

The grave was restored by the Lignum Vitae Club, an association of Jamaican women in London, and by the British Commonwealth Nurses' War Memorial Fund. These two organisations, with the support of the UK Jamaican Nurses' Association, which took initial responsibility for the upkeep of the grave, held a re-consecration ceremony in 1973. Sir Laurence Lindo, the then High Commissioner for Jamaica, was among those present at the service.

"She has indeed, I assure you, and with great disinterestedness," replied Soyer. "While I was there this morning, she was dressing a poor Land Transport Corps man, who had received a severe contusion on the head. In order to strengthen his courage for the process, as she said, she made him a glass of strong brandy and water, not charging him anything for it; and I hear that she has done this repeatedly." "I am sure she has done much good," Florence replied.

Soyer (1857) makes several mentions of a daughter named Sarah/Sally Seacole and how she referred to Mary as "Mother". In notes of conversations Florence had with her sister Parthenope, cited by Mark Bostridge (2004), there is mention of Mary having an illegitimate 14-year-old daughter, the father a Colonel Bunbury. Jane Robinson's research (2005) appears to rule out these possibilities, but Florence may have believed the rumours. Robinson's (2005) own investigation of the undated documentation of conversations between Florence and Parthenope (Claydon House Trust) reveals even more negative comments. Florence refers to Mary as a "woman of bad character" who kept a "bad house" and who had to be discouraged from visiting a sick Florence in Balaklava in order to "quack" her. Bostridge also records a further reference, which would certainly account for Florence's possible resentment against Mary: "Seacole had won the protection of Nightingale's great adversary, Dr John Hall, Inspector-General of Hospitals in the Crimea, who had given Seacole 'his sanction' to prescribe her medicines."

In this same year, Trinidadian writer Therese Mills (1973) included a chapter about Mary Seacole in a children's book about famous West Indians.

1975   One of the first articles about Mary Seacole in a British nursing journal was published, written by J Elise Gordon.

1980   Brent Library Service launched a touring exhibition, *Roots in Britain*, produced by Ziggi Alexander and Audrey Dewjee. It featured hundreds of illustrations depicting the lives of earlier black settlers. The display included information on Mary Seacole and, "from all over the British Isles the exhibition comments books arrived with one recurring request – additional information on Mary Seacole".

1981   Alexander and Dewjee became involved in a memorial service and procession to the grave of Mary Seacole, which was held on 14 May to mark the centenary of Mary's death. They also published an article about Mary in *History Today* (Alexander and Dewjee, 1981). A Mary Seacole Society was formed in Leamington Spa (Tywang, 2004).

1982   Alexander and Dewjee published the pamphlet: *Mary Seacole. Jamaican national heroine and "doctress" in the Crimean War*.

1983   The Friends of Mary Seacole was founded and was later renamed the Mary Seacole Memorial Association. It took over responsibility for the upkeep of Mary's grave and organising an annual memorial service and wreath-laying ceremony (Tywang, 2004).

1984   A new edition of Mary Seacole's autobiography (Alexander and Dewjee, 1984) received extensive media coverage, including in the nursing press (Iveson-Iveson, 1984; Watson, 1984; Smith, 1984).

Learning about Seacole's story

Some nurses are angry that they were not taught about Mary Seacole alongside Florence Nightingale (Anionwu, 2003; Bassett, 1992; Crawford, 1992). "The next generation should receive information about her routinely, just as they do about Florence Nightingale. If people want to know the history of who has contributed to the nursing profession they need to know that, in her time, Mary Seacole was recognised in a similar way to Florence Nightingale. And no one should leave a three-year nursing course without knowing that," (Pearce, 2004).

In an article by a nursing tutor (Bassett, 1992), the writer recalls his efforts over three years to track down Mary Seacole's autobiography (which had been reprinted in 1984). He discovers that the RCN Library did not have a copy, but manages to borrow it from the British Library.

We hope that nursing educationalists adopt a more systematic approach, and right this imbalance - both Victorian nurses offer important insights into nursing practice. Students are encouraged to read Florence Nightingale's *Notes on Nursing* and *Wonderful Adventures of Mrs Seacole in Many Lands*.

School pupils already benefit from such an approach - many more young people than adults are aware of Mary. This is because the Qualifications and Curriculum Authority included both Seacole and Nightingale in the National Curriculum in History, Key Stage 2, under the section for Victorian Britain (DfEE, 1999).

Sources of information
It is important that students recognise that Mary, like Florence, was a complex human being and both had their own frailties. Mary Seacole should not be viewed as a saintly figure. But there are now several detailed critiques about her life which are essential reading to develop a deeper understanding. They provide an insight into how Mary was perceived by others, and the likely opinions that

In September, the Yorkshire Television programme *First Tuesday* included a feature *Mary Seacole, a notable nurse*. The 11-minute documentary included interviews with Ziggi Alexander and several black nurses who recounted their experiences of racism in the NHS (Tywang, 2004).

1985   The Greater London Council (GLC) marked Mary Seacole's former home at 157 George Street, London W1, with a blue plaque. Since the building's demolition in 1998, a planning dispute has delayed the plaque's transfer to another former residence, 14 Soho Square not far from Oxford Street (Sakula, 1998; Agnew, 2005).

1989   Oval House theatre in London puts on Michael Bath's play *Black Nightingale: the true story of Mary Seacole*.

1990   The Jamaican Order of Merit was bestowed posthumously on Mary Seacole (*The Jamaican Gazette Extraordinary*, 1990).

Ziggi Alexander makes reference to a letter from Florence Nightingale to her brother-in-law Sir Harry Verney (dated 5 August 1870), where Florence makes clear her very mixed views about Mary Seacole (see page 31) (Alexander, 1990).

1991   A postal stamp featuring Mary Seacole was issued in Jamaica to commemorate a meeting of the International Council of Nurses *(The Times Diary*, 1991).

1992   A Mary Seacole Exhibition was opened in April, organised by Black Cultural Archives in collaboration with the Florence Nightingale Museum (Walker, 2005).

1994   The Mary Seacole Leadership Award was launched by the Department of Health to recognise the contribution of black and minority ethnic nurses. The scholarship, covering a 10-year period, was developed after: "A number of notable dignitaries wrote to the Prime Minister and suggested that some public recognition should be made in Mary Seacole's name to mark the contribution she made to the war effort in the Crimea" (DH, 2000). The award of £25,000 to cover a year's project for one individual, is administered by the

she held, covering topics such as gender, identity, race, class, war and foreigners (Alexander and Dewjee, 1984; McKenna, 1997; Hawthorne, 2000; Frederick, 2003; Kavalski, 2003; Salih, 2005; Rappaport, 2005; Robinson, 2005). Some of these appraisals are not always flattering. An interesting example of one of Mary's robust point of views is: "Some people, indeed, have called me quite a female Ulysses. I believe that they intended it as a complement; but from my experience of the Greeks, I do not consider it a flattering one." Nevertheless there is a remarkable body of evidence demonstrating that Victorian contemporaries did enthusiastically acknowledge her nursing expertise, commitment and determination.

Royal College of Nursing working with the Royal College of Midwives, the Community Practitioners and Health Visitors Association and UNISON.

1996   The Mary Seacole Research Centre, De Montfort University, Leicester, was established by Mel Chevannes, Professor of Nursing (Mary Seacole Research Centre, 1999).

1998   The Mary Seacole Centre for Nursing Practice at Thames Valley University, London, was founded by Elizabeth Anionwu, Professor of Nursing (Pearce, 2004).

2000   The UKCC (now the Nursing and Midwifery Council) named a room after Mary Seacole, "in recognition of the UKCC's commitment to valuing the diversity of the professions which it regulates and the society which it serves" (NMC).

In September, BBC Knowledge TV digital channel broadcast a 30-minute documentary about Mary Seacole produced by October Films (Carpenter, 2000). Following a three-year campaign for a wider showing of the programme, BBC2 agree to transmit it in March 2005 (*Nursing Standard*, 2004).

A *Mary Seacole* opera was performed at the Royal Opera House, Covent Garden in October (Taylor, 2000). Richard Chew composed the music, the librettist was SuAndi and the singers included Hyacinth Nicholls and Wills Morgan.

2003   Former London MP Clive Soley, now Lord Soley, launched an appeal in November to erect a statue of Mary Seacole in central London (Duffin, 2004). Meanwhile, a Mary Seacole musical was showcased at the Greenwich Theatre (www. maryseacole.co.uk).

2004   150th anniversary of the British involvement in the Crimean War (Kerr et al., 2000; Ponting, 2004).

In a national Internet poll, Mary Seacole was voted the Greatest Black Briton – the news received extensive media coverage (Taylor, 2004). Tens of thousands of people voted and Mary came out ahead of historical figures such

A student perspective

Pamela Bennie, Nursing Student, University of Wales, Bangor
RCN ANS Executive Committee member for Wales

I feel honoured to be asked as a student nurse how Mary Seacole continues to inspire me. It is because of Mary Seacole's desire and determination to care for soldiers in the Crimean War that I am able to question and justify why I chose nursing as a profession.

The significant reason for my choice of nursing was my desire to care for people from a wide range of backgrounds. I felt that in the health care profession, having a holistic view meant that I could see everyone's need for clinical care, regardless of their colour, creed, nationality or religious beliefs. My priority at all times will be to deliver the very best care.

Nursing is a complex and yet very rewarding career to have. Nursing students face immense pressure to pass both theoretical and practical examinations. I feel I have to put in double the effort my non-nursing colleagues do in order to attain the same grades. There are great expectations when we are on clinical practice placements; competences must be achieved, but it can be very hard when faced with real life situations. I hope I can always act within the code of professional conduct, and my concern is always the benefit of the patient, for whom I came into nursing.

I have read Mary Seacole's trials, tribulations and successes, and being able to recollect how difficult providing care was for her helps me continue to strive for high standards of care and compassion against all odds. Her concern, like me, was the patient. Mary Seacole will always continue to inspire my profession because of her ability to overcome many obstacles to deliver care in the most difficult conditions. She is an excellent role model for all student and qualified nurses. We, like Mary, are obligated to deliver good nursing care.

as Olaudah Equiano, writer and political activist (c1745-1797), and present day celebrities including singer Dame Shirley Bassey.

The Mary Seacole Memorial Statue Appeal was the RCN President's chosen charity at RCN Congress 2004, where the inaugural annual Mary Seacole Lecture was given by Professor Elizabeth Anionwu of the Mary Seacole Centre for Nursing Practice, Thames Valley University (www.rcn.org. uk; *Nursing Standard*, 2004a).

The Department of Health launched a new Mary Seacole Development Award covering a five-year period, providing £6,500 to each of four nurses, midwives and health visitors. Four nursing unions expressed concern at the significantly lower amount now presented to each winner compared with the earlier award (*Nursing Standard*, 2004b).

The University of Wolverhampton opened its Mary Seacole School of Health Building (*New Insight*, 2004).

2005 The 200th anniversary of the year of Mary Seacole's birth.

The Home Office names one of its new offices in Victoria the Seacole Building.

The London School of Hygiene and Tropical Medicine names a Board Room after Mary Seacole.

The Florence Nightingale Museum launches a year-long Mary Seacole Bicentenary London 2005 exhibition.

In June, C4 television broadcast Mary Seacole: The Real Angel of the Crimea, an hour-long documentary and reconstruction of her life.

Mary Seacole's relevance today

Mary Seacole's resolution, skills and compassion are relevant to all nurses and midwives today. She has widespread appeal to many different groups, including historians, women travellers and the military, but especially:

- all today's nurses. Mary provided the sick and injured with a place of refuge. She listened to their needs and showed care and compassion; she also undertook diagnoses and minor surgery, and supplied medicines - much like her modern successors
- middle-aged and older women. Let's not forget that Mary was 50 when she left to nurse in the Crimean War, and did not let age stand in her way
- black and minority ethnic nurses. It's not surprising that Mary holds a special place in the hearts of many black and minority ethnic nurses, and the wider public, for although she faced discrimination, she did not allow it to crush her. "By emphasizing her 'strong-mindedness', she further counters prevailing views of black dependency. ...Seacole also testifies to the strength of her own response to racial hostility..." (Hawthorne, 2000).

The words of a former Editor-in-Chief of the *Journal of Advanced Nursing*, James Smith (1997), make a heartening conclusion. He identified Mary Seacole as one of several British nurses whose legacy to the profession should be remembered: "Alas, their names and contributions to the professional development of nursing are almost in danger of being erased from the collective memory of the nursing profession. That should be checked. The same fate befell the outstanding work of Mary Seacole, a nineteenth century black British nurse. Fortunately she has been brought back to the notice of the profession again. She is a marvellous role model for today's nurses – black and non-black alike."

References

Agnew T (2005) Seacole blue plaque plan delayed by building row, *Nursing Standard*, Vol 19, No. 23, p.4.

Alexander Z (1990) Let it lie upon the table: the status of black women's biography in the UK, *Gender & History*, Vol 2 (No 1), pp.22-33.

Alexander Z and Dewjee A (1981) Blacks in Britain: Mary Seacole, *History Today*, Vol 31, Issue: 9, p. 45.

Alexander Z and Dewjee A (1982) *Mary Seacole. Jamaican national heroine and "doctress" in the Crimean War*, London: Brent Library Service.

Alexander Z and Dewjee A (1984) Editors' introduction, pp.9-45. *Wonderful Adventures of Mrs Seacole in many lands*, Bristol: Falling Wall Press.

Anionwu E N (2003) It's time for a statue of Mary Seacole, *Nursing Times*, Vol 99, No. 32, p.17.

Bassett C (1992) Viewpoint: Mary Seacole: the forgotten founder, *Nursing Standard*, Vol 6 (31), pp.44-45.

Black C V (1943) *Living names in Jamaica's history* (contains a biographical sketch of Mary Seacole), Kingston: Jamaican Welfare.

Bostridge M (2004) Ministering on distant shores, *The Guardian*, Saturday Review, 14 February, p.7.

Carpenter S (2000) The forgotten angel of the Crimea, *The Times*, Times 2 Analysis, 4 September, pp.12-13.

Claydon House Trust collection, MS Nightingale 110. Undated. (The author is grateful to Jane Robinson for providing additional information about these papers.)

Cootes-Peterkin E (1961) From suitcase …. the story of Mary Seacole House, *The Jamaican Nurse*. Reprinted in The Jamaican Nurse, August 1986, Vol 25 (1, 2, 3), pp.55-56.

Cootes-Peterkin E (June 1961a) Happy birthday Mary Seacole House, *The Jamaican Nurse*. Reprinted in *The Jamaican Nurse*, August 1986, Vol 25 (1, 2, 3), p.58.

Crawford P (1992) The other lady with the lamp, *Nursing Times*, Vol 88 (11), pp.56-58.

Department of Education and Employment (1999) *History. The National Curriculum for England: key stages 1-3*, London: DfEE & QCA. Available online via: www.nc.uk.net

Department of Health (2000) *Black and ethnic nurses, midwives and health visitors leading change. A report of the Mary Seacole leadership award – the first five years*, London: DH.

Dossey B M, Selanders L C, Beck D M and Attewell A (2005) *Florence Nightingale today: healing, leadership, global action*, Silverspring (MD): American Nurses Association.

Duffin C (2004) Seacole's story in stone, *Nursing Standard*, Vol 18 (42), p.7. See also www.maryseacoleappeal.org.uk for further details about the Mary Seacole Memorial Statue Appeal.

Florence Nightingale Museum website: www.florence-nightingale.co.uk

Frederick R (2003) Creole performance in Wonderful Adventures of Mrs Seacole in Many Lands, *Gender & History*, 15 (3), pp. 487-506.

Fryer P (1984) *Staying power. The history of black people in Britain*, London: Pluto Press.

Getty Museum: www.getty.edu/art/ collections/objects/o1522.html

Gill G (2004) *Nightingales. The story of Florence Nightingale and her remarkable family*, London: Hodder & Stoughton.

Gordon J E (1975) Mary Seacole - a forgotten nurse heroine of the Crimea, *Midwife, Health Visitor & Community Nurse*, 11 (2), pp.47-50.

Gustafson M (1996) Mary Seacole, the Florence Nightingale of Jamaica, *Christian Nurse International*, 12(4), p.9.

Hawthorne E J (2000) Self-writing, literary traditions and post-emancipation identity: The case of Mary Seacole, *Biography: an Interdisciplinary Quarterly*, 23, no.2, pp.309-331.

Iveson-Iveson J (1984) A pin to see a peep show, *Nursing Mirror*, Vol 158 No 13, p.36.

Jamaican Nurse (1973) Mary Seacole honoured in London in ceremony of reconstruction, *Jamaican Nurse*, Vol 13 (3) December, reprinted in *Jamaican Nurse* (1981), Vol 21 (2), p.15.

The Jamaican Gazette Extraordinary (1990), 3 August, Vol, CXIII No. 30-1A. This is an official Jamaican government document, containing the announcement of the award of the Jamaican Order of Merit to Mary Seacole.

Kavalski E (2003) Notions of voluntary identity and citizenship in the *Wonderful Adventures of Mrs Seacole in Many Lands, Jouvert* 7(2) accessed online via: http://social.chass.ncsu.edu/jouvert/v7i2/kavals.htm

Kerr P, Pye P, Cherfas T, Gold M and Mulvihill M et al (2000) *The Crimean War*, London: Channel 4 Books.

Mary Seacole Musical details: www.maryseacole.co.uk

Mary Seacole Research Centre (1999) *1998-1999 annual report*, Leicester: De Montfort University.

McGuffie G (2004) Personal communication by Elizabeth Anionwu with Gavin McGuffie, archivist, *Guardian and Observer* Archive and Visitor Centre. The notice of the death of Mary Seacole was featured on 23 May 1881, p.7, column 7.

McKenna B (1997) "Fancies of exclusive possession": Validation and discussion in Mary Seacole's England and Caribbean. *Philological Quarterly*, Vol 76, Part 2, pp. 219-239.

Messmer P R and Parchment Y (1996) The Florence Nightingale of Jamaica - Mary Seacole, nurse pioneer, *Reflections*, 22(4):26, 4th quarter.

Mills T (1973) *Great West Indians: life stories for young readers*. London: Longmans Caribbean Ltd.

National Library of Jamaica: www.nlj.org.jm/index.htm

New Insight (2004) Official opening for Mary Seacole Building, *staff letter*, issue 10, December, University of Wolverhampton. www.wlv.ac.uk/newinsight

Nightingale F (1860) *Notes on nursing: what it is, and what it is not*, London: Harrison and Sons.

Nightingale F (1870) *Letter from Florence Nightingale to Sir Harry Verney* (dated 5 August 1870), Wellcome Library for the History and Understanding of Medicine, MS 9004.

Nursing and Midwifery Council. See: www.nmc-uk.org/nmc/main/home/ 23PortlandPlace-HomeOfTheNmc.html

Nursing Mirror (1977) In loving memory. A woman of enormous courage (tribute to J Elise Gordon), *Nursing Mirror*, Vol 144 (6), pp.33, 35.

Nursing Standard (2004) News in brief, *Nursing Standard*, Vol 19 (13), p.8.

Nursing Standard (2004a) RCN Congress: we can still learn from Mary Seacole, *Nursing Standard*, Vol 18(36), p.7.

Nursing Standard (2004b) Unions plead for Seacole boost, *Nursing Standard*, Vol 19 (8), p.4.

Nursing Standard (2005) Seacole portrait takes rightful place, *Nursing Standard*, Vol 19 (18), p.4.

Pearce L (2004) Tribute to a visionary, *Nursing Standard*, Vol 19 (4), pp.16-17.

Ponting C (2004) *The Crimean War. The truth behind the myth*, London: Chatto and Windus. See also www.crimeanwar.org

Portrait: Examples of coverage on 11 January 2005 of the discovery of a portrait of Mary Seacole include: Reynolds R, Crimea heroine who turned up in a car boot sale, p.9, *The Daily Telegraph*; Alberge D, Black heroine emerges from cover- up, p.28, *The Times*; Higgins C, Historic portrait of Crimean war nurse unveiled, p.9, *The Guardian*.

Public Record Office, ref: WO 25/264. Reference kindly supplied by Paul Kerr, October Films. Elizabeth Anionwu is also grateful to Ziggi Alexander for providing details of her 1990 paper that first cited this reference. London: PRO. www.pro.gov.uk

Punch, 6 December 1856, page 221.

Rappaport H (2005) The invitation that never came, *History Today,* Vol 55 (02), pp.9-15.

Robinson J (2005) *Mary Seacole - the charismatic black nurse who became a heroine of the Crimea*, London: Constable.

Robinson J (2005a) Personal communication with Elizabeth Anionwu, showing this information in Jane Robinson's book (page 30) is taken from the baptism registration dated 18 September 1803: "Edwin Horatio Hamilton Seacole was baptized, and probably born, in Prittlewell, Essex, in 1803."

Rogers J A (originally privately published in 1947, reprinted in 1996) *World's great men of color*. Volume 11 New York: Touchstone/ Simon and Schuster.

Royal College of Nursing. See: www.rcn. org.uk/downloads/congress2004/bulletin/ tuesday.pdf

Sakula A (1998) Mary Seacole (1805-1881): 157 George Street, W1, in plaques on London houses of medical-historical interest, *Journal of medical biography*, Vol 6 (3), p.148.

Salih S (2005) Editor's introduction, pp.xv-l *Wonderful Adventures of Mrs Seacole in Many Lands*, London: Penguin Classics.

Seacole M (1857) *Wonderful Adventures of Mrs Seacole in Many Lands*, London: James Blackwood. See also Alexander and Dewjee (1984), and Salih (2005).

Seacole M (1876) *Will* (copy viewed courtesy of Paul Kerr, October Films). In Mary's will dated 2 September 1876, she refers to herself as the widow of Edwin Horatio Seacole and bequeaths to "His Serene Highness the Count Gleichen the diamond ring given to my late husband by his Godfather Viscount Nelson".

Seaton H J (2002) *Another Florence Nightingale? The rediscovery of Mary Seacole* at www.victorianweb.org/history/crimea/seacole.html

Seivwright M (1961) Mary Seacole: the Florence Nightingale of Jamaica, *The Jamaican Nurse*: 1(2) 8-9. Reprinted in *The Jamaican Nurse* (August 1986) Vol 25: (1, 2, 3), pp.49-50.

Small H (1998) *Florence Nightingale. Avenging angel*, London: Constable.

Smith J P (1984) Mary Jane Seacole 1805-1881: a black British nurse, *Journal of Advanced Nursing*, 9(5), pp.427-48.

Smith J P (1997) Liminal nurses urgently needed for the challenges ahead, *Journal of Advanced Nursing* Sep: 26(3), pp.437–38.

Soyer A (1995 with introductions by Michael Barthorp and Elizabeth Ray, originally published 1857) *A culinary campaign*, Lewes: Southover Press.

Taylor K (2000) Labour of love, *The Voice*: 18 September, p.9.

Taylor M (2004) Nurse is greatest black Briton, *The Guardian* 10 February, p.5. For online summary of, and links to further media coverage, visit: www.100greatblackbritons.com/news.html

The Times Diary (1991) Stamp of success, *The Times*, 22 July, p.14.

Thompson A M C (1968) *A bibliography of nursing literature 1859-1961*, London: The Library Association for the Royal College of Nursing and the National Council of Nurses of the United Kingdom in association with King Edward's Hospital Fund for London.

Thompson A M C (1974) *A bibliography of nursing literature 1961- 1970*, London: The Library Association for the Royal College of Nursing and the National Council of Nurses of the United Kingdom in association with King Edward's Hospital Fund for London.

Trollope A (originally published 1859, reprinted 1999) *The West Indies and the Spanish Main*, New York: Carroll and Graf Publishers Inc.

Tulloch E (1971) Historical perspectives of nursing in Jamaica, *International Nursing Review*, Vol 18 (1), pp.49-57.

Tywang M (2004) Personal communication by Elizabeth Anionwu with Sister Monica Tywang, former Chairperson of the Mary Seacole Memorial Association and Chaplain of West Indians (1976-1992).

University of the West Indies, Mary Seacole Hall (1985) *Handbook – academic year 1985-86*, Jamaica: University of West Indies. See also: www.mona.uwi.edu/halls/seacole/

Vernon C (1969) The Florence Nightingale of Jamaica, *The Jamaican Nurse*, Vol 9 (3), p.19. Reprinted in *The Jamaican Nurse*, August 1986, Vol 25 (1, 2, 3), pp.47-51.

Walker S (2005) Personal communication by Elizabeth Anionwu with Sam Walker, Director of the Black Cultural Archives in London. The Mary Seacole exhibition, aimed at schools, was a collaborative project undertaken with the Florence Nightingale Museum and toured the UK for several months in 1992.

Walsh F (1985) *A bibliography of nursing literature (the Holdings of the Royal College of Nursing 1971-1975)*, London: The Library Association.

Walsh F (1986) *A bibliography of nursing literature (the Holdings of the Royal College of Nursing 1976-1980)*, London: The Library Association.

Watson C (1984) Hidden from history, *Nursing Times*, News Focus, 10 October, Vol 80 (41), pp.16-17.

Williams M (2005) Personal communication by Marjorie Williams with Elizabeth Anionwu, following a contact with Kingston Public Hospital.

Wilson A N (2003) *The Victorians*, London: Arrow Books (originally published by Hutchinson, 2002).

Woodham-Smith C (1950) *Florence Nightingale*, London: Constable.

Young R (2004) Crimea nurse is greatest black Briton, *The Times*, 10 February, p.26.

Web resources

www.maryseacole.com
Website of the Mary Seacole Centre for Nursing Practice, Thames Valley University. Contains detailed information relating to Mary Seacole.

www.maryseacoleappeal.org.uk/
Website of the Mary Seacole Memorial Statue Appeal.

www.100greatblackbritons.com
Website of 100 Great Black Britons in which Mary Seacole was voted number one.

www4.umdnj.edu/camlbweb/blacknurses
Black nurses in history. This is a guide from the USA-based UMDNJ and Coriell Research Library.

www.suite101.com/article.cfm/crimean_war/110329
A series of five articles about Mary Seacole written by military historian John Barham between 6 August and 26 November 2004.

www.florence-nightingale.co.uk/
Website of the Florence Nightingale Museum, London.